simple & easy
calorie counter

CAFE LATTE PRESS

ISBN: 9798567107577

SIMPLE & EASY CALORIE COUNTER

SUPER LOW CALORIE FOODS

Quick, easy-to-scan guide to the best super low calorie options from all food groups, meals & snacks listed

MEALS

FOOD GROUPS

super
low calorie
foods

SUPER LOW CALORIE FOODS

VEGETABLES

Arugula (1 cup) = 3 cal

Asparagus (1 cup) = 27 cal

Beets (1 cup) = 59 cal

Bok Choy (1 cup) = 9 cal

Broccoli (1 cup) = 31 cal

Brussel Sprouts (1 cup) = 38 cal

Cabbage (1 cup) = 22 cal

Carrots (1 cup) = 53cal

Cauliflower (1 cup) = 25 cal

Celery (1 cup) = 18 cal

Cucumber (1 cup) = 16 cal

Eggplant (1 cup) = 20 cal

Fennel (1 cup) = 27 cal

Garlic (1 clove) = 5 cal

Green Beans (1 cup) = 35 cal

Kale (1 cup) = 34 cal

Lettuce, Iceberg (1 cup) = 10 cal

Lettuce (1 cup) = 5 cal

Mushrooms (1 cup) = 15 cal

Mustard Greens (1 cup) = 15 cal

Okra (1 cup) = 33 cal

Onions (1 cup) = 46 cal

Peppers (1 cup) = 46 cal

Pumpkin (1 cup) = 30 cal

Radishes (1 cup) = 19 cal

Spinach (1 cup) = 7 cal

Tomatoes (1 cup) = 27 cal

Turnips (1 cup) = 36 cal

White Mushrooms (1 cup) = 15 cal

Watercress (1 cup) = 4 cal

Zucchini (1 cup) = 18 cal

SUPER LOW CALORIE FOODS

FRUITS

Apple (1 med apple) = 57 cal

Apricot (1 fruit) = 17 cal

Blackberries (1 cup) = 62 cal

Blueberries (1 cup)= = 85 cal

Cantaloupe (1 cup) = 55 cal

Cherries (1 cup) = 77 cal

Clementines (1 fruit) = 35 cal

Cranberries (1 cup) = 46 cal

Grapes (1 cup) = 62 cal

Honeydew Melon (1 cup) = 61 cal

Grapefruit (1 fruit) = 97 cal

Kiwi (1 fruit) = 49 cal

Lemon & Lime (1 fluid oz.) = 4 cal

Mango (1 cup) = 100 cal (1 fruit) = 200 cal

Nectarine (1 fruit) = 67 cal

Orange (1 fruit) = 62 cal

Papaya (1 cup) = 55 cal

Pears (1 fruit) = 100 cal

Peach (1 fruit) = 59 cal

Pineapple (1 cup) = 82 cal

Plum (1 fruit) = 30 cal

Raspberries (1 cup) = 65 cal

Rhubarb (1 cup) = 11 cal

Strawberries (1 cup) = 50 cal

Tangerine (1 fruit) = 47 cal

Watermelon (1 cup, diced) = 46 cal

SUPER LOW CALORIE FOODS

MEAT & POULTRY

Chicken Breast (no skin, 3 oz) = 140 cal

Chicken Meatballs (3 meatballs) = 130 cal

Pork Tenderloin (3 oz cut) = 135 cal

Turkey (slice, deli) = 28 cal

Turkey, Roast Turkey (3 oz) = 125 cal

Veggie meatballs (3 meatballs) = 100 cal

FISH & SEAFOOD

Cod, Baked (1 fillet) = 190 cal

Mahi Mahi, Grilled (1 steak fillet) = 135 cal

Scallops (5 sm scallops) = 26 cal

Salmon, Baked/Steamed (1 fillet) = 120 cal

Tilapia Baked (1 fillet) = 110 cal

DAIRY & EGGS

Cottage Cheese, Fat Free (1/2 cup) = 53 cal

Eggs (1 egg) = 72 cal

Egg Whites (3 tbsp = 1 egg) = 25 cal

Milk, Skim,1% Low-fat or Nonfat (1/2 cup) = 51 cal (1 cup) = 102 cal

Mozzarella Cheese, Part Skim (1 oz /1 slice) = 70 cal

Yogurt, Nonfat (1 cup) = 100 cal, (w/fruit) 110-120 cal

NUTS & BEANS

Almond Milk, unsweetened (1 cup) = 38 cal

Chestnuts (1 oz) = 63 cal

Chia Seeds (1 tbsp) = 70 cal

SUPER LOW CALORIE FOODS

GRAINS

Crackers, Water (4 crackers) = 60 cal

Oatmeal (1/2 cup, cooked) = 150 cal

Popcorn (1 cup) = 31 cal

Rice Cake (1 rice cake) = 35 cal

Shirataki Noodles (3 oz) = 5 cal

Wild Rice, cooked (3/4 cup) = 125 cal

SOUPS

Broth (chk-bf-vg,1 cup) = 7-12 cal

Chicken Noodle Soup (1 cup) = 87 cal

Chicken Rice Soup (1 cup) = 60 cal

Fish Soup (1 cup) = 105 cal

Vegetable Soup (1 cup) = 80 cal

DRINKS

Coffee, Black (1 cup) = 2 cal

Coffee, Latte Nonfat, w/skim milk (1 cup) = 70 cal

Juice, Orange Juice, Trop 50 (1 cup) = 50 cal

Herbal tea (1 cup) = 0-5 cal

Tea, Green Tea, brewed(1 cup) = 2 cal

Water, carbonated (1 cup) = 0 cal

Water (1 cup) = 0 cal

SUPER LOW CALORIE FOODS

DESSERTS

Angel Food Cake (1 piece) = 110 cal

Applesauce, unsweetened (1 cup) = 50 cal

Fruit Salad w/grapes (1 cup) = 74 cal

Parfait, Homemade Parfait, yogurt/fruit/honey (1 parfait) = 150 cal

SNACKS

Angel Food Cake (1 piece) = 110 cal

Applesauce, unsweetened (1 cup) = 50 cal

Cheese & Water Crackers, w/mozz cheese (4 crackers, 1 oz Mozz) = 137 cal

French Fries, Oven Baked Fries, from frozen, (10 fries) = 99 cal

Fruit Salad w/grapes (1 cup) = 74 cal

Graham Crackers, Lowfat (1 full cracker sheet) = 60 cal

Melba Toast (3 toasts) = 60 cal

Parfait, Homemade Parfait, yogurt/fruit/honey (1 parfait) = 150 cal

Pickles (1 pickle) = 5 cal

Rice Cake (1 cake)= 15 cal

String cheese, Light (1 mozzarella cheese stick) = 50 cal

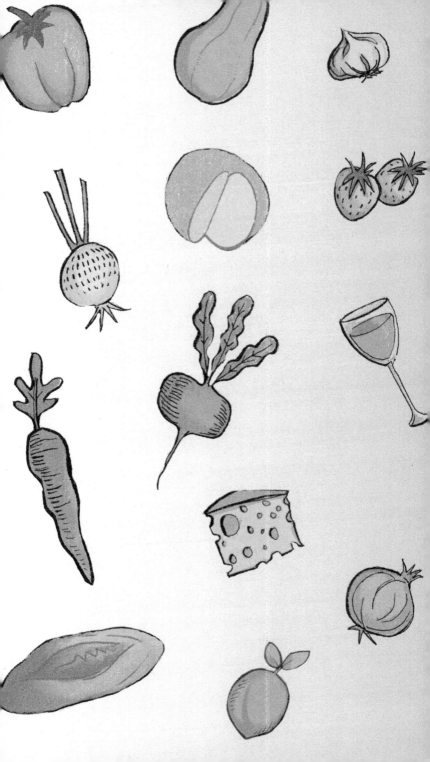

meals

MEALS

BREAKFAST

Avocado Toast (1 piece) = 200 cal

Bacon (1 slice) = 50 cal (2 slices) = 100 cal

Banana (1 med fruit) = 105 cal

Bagel, plain (1 med bagel) = 250 cal

Bagel, plain w/cream cheese (1 med bagel) = 370 cal

Breakfast Burrito, Sausage, Egg & Cheese (1 sandwich) = 500 cal

Breakfast Sandwich, Egg & Cheese (1 sandwich) = 340 cal

Breakfast Sandwich, Sausage, Egg & Cheese (1 sandwich) = 500 cal

Breakfast Sandwich, Turkey Bacon, Egg White (1 sandwich) = 210 cal

Cereal, regular, plain w/1% milk (1 cup) = 170 cal

Cereal, Crispix w/1% milk (1 cup) = 160

Cereal, Rice Krispies w/1% milk (1 cup) = 160

Cereal, Raisin Bran w/1% milk (1 cup) = 238 cal

Croissant, Plain Butter (1 croissant) = 230 cal

Croissant, Chocolate (1 croissant) = 340 cal

Croissant, Almond (1 croissant) = 420 cal

Croissant, Ham & Swiss Cheese (1 croissant) = 320 cal

Danish, Cinnamon Bun (1 danish) = 330 cal

Donut, Cream filled donut (1 med donut) = 343 cal

Danish, Danish pastry (1 danish) = 270 cal

Donut, Glazed donut (1 med donut) = 300 cal

Donut, Jelly donut (1 med donut) = 289 cal

Donut, Plain old fashioned donut (1 med donut) = 270 cal

Eggs Benedict (2 eggs) = 553 cal

Eggs, Boiled (1 egg) = 78 cal

Eggs, Omelette, Ham & Cheese (2 eggs) = 300cal

MEALS

BREAKFAST

Eggs, Omelette, Spinach, Mushroom, Tomato w/fresh fruit (2 eggs) = 330 cal

Eggs, Omelette, Veggies + Cheeses (2 eggs) = 495 cal

Eggs, Scrambled (1 egg) = 90 cal, (2 eggs) = 198 cal

Eggs, Sunnyside Up (1 egg) = 90 cal (2 eggs) = 180 cal

Egg Whites (3 tbsp = 1 egg) = 25 cal (6 tbsp = 2 eggs) = 50 cal

Hash Browns (1/2 cup) = 210 cal (1 cup) = 413 cal

French Toast, buttered (2 slices) = 356 cal

Fruit Bowl, mixed fruit (1/2 cup) = 70 cal (1 cup) = 124 cal

Fruit Salad w/grapes (1/2 cup) = 37 cal, (1 cup) = 74 cal

Oatmeal, cooked w/1% milk (1/2 cup) = 210 cal

Muffin, Blueberry (lg muffin) = 426 cal

Muffin, Banana Walnut (lg muffin) = 589 cal

Pancake, butter, syrup (lg pancake) = 520 cal

Pancakes, butter, syrup (3 med pancakes) = 780 cal

Sausage, Breakfast Sausage, pork (3 sm links) = 180 cal

Sausage, Turkey Sausage (3 sm links) = 100 cal

Scone, plain (lg scone) = 400 cal

Scone, w/blueberries (lg scone) = 420 cal

Scone, w/raisins (lg scone) = 450 cal

Toast, Wheat, buttered (1 slice) = 169 cal, (2 slices) = 338 cal

Toast, White, buttered (1 slice) = 169 cal, (2 slices) = 338 cal

Waffles, w/butter (1 waffle, 7") = 250 cal, (2 waffles) = 500 cal

Waffles, Belgian w/strawberries, whipped cream, syrup (1 waffle) = 540 cal

Yogurt, Plain (1 cup) = 90-110 cal, w/fruit = 110-150 cal

Yogurt, Greek Yogurt, Plain (1 cup) = 100-130 cal, w/fruit = 110-140 cal

Yogurt, Light, Non Fat Yogurt (1 cup) = 80-110 cal, w/fruit = 100-120 cal

MEALS

LUNCH / DINNER

BBQ Ribs (1/2 rack, 6 ribs) = 762 cal

Beans, Baked Beans (1/2 cup) = 191 cal (1 cup) = 382 cal

Beans, Black Beans, boiled w/salt (1/2 cup) = 114 cal, (1 cup) = 227 cal

Beans, Pinto Beans, boiled w/salt (1/2 cup) = 123 cal, (1 cup) = 245 cal

Beans, Refried Beans (1/2 cup) = 110 cal, (1 cup) = 220 cal

Black Beans & Rice (1 cup meal) = 244 cal

Beef, Brisket (3 oz) = 296 cal

Beef, Ground Beef, hamburger meat, sautéed, 80% lean (3 oz) = 200 cal

Beef, Hamburger Steak (1 serving) = 296 cal

Beef Stew, homemade, (1 cup) = 267 cal (1 bowl) = 535 cal

Beef Stroganoff (1 cup) = 300 cal (1 plate) = 600 cal

Buffalo Wings w/dip (order of 5 wings) = 1200 cal

Burger, Cheeseburger w/toppings (reg size) = 400 cal, (lg size) = 550-700 cal

Burger, Hamburger w/toppings (reg size) = 300 cal, (lg size) = 400-500 cal

Burger, Veggie Burger w/toppings, restaurant (lg size) = 350-550 cal

Burger, Veggie Burger, Black Bean veggie burger, (just 1 patty) = 120 cal, (as burger) = 320 cal

Burger, Veggie Burger, Trader Joe's Quinoa Cowboy Veggie Burger, (just 1 patty) = 180 cal, (as burger) = 380 cal

Burger, Veggie Burger, Trader Joe's Vegetable Masala burger, (just 1 patty) = 140 cal, (as burger) = 340 cal

Burrito, Chicken Burrito w/toppings, Chipotle (1 burrito) = 1450 cal

Burrito, Shredded Pork Burrito w/toppings, Chipotle (1 burrito) = 1480 cal

Burrito, Steak Burrito w/toppings, Chipotle (1 burrito) = 1420 cal

Burrito, Veggie Burrito w/toppings, Chipotle (1 burrito) = 1055 cal

Burrito Bowl, Chicken Burrito Bowl w/toppings, Chipotle (1 burrito bowl) = 1115 cal

MEALS

LUNCH / DINNER

Burrito Bowl, Shredded Pork Bowl w/toppings, Chipotle (1 burrito bowl) = 1145 cal

Burrito Bowl, Steak Burrito Bowl w/toppings, Chipotle (1 burrito bowl) = 1085 cal

Burrito Bowl, Veggie Burrito Bowl w/toppings, Chipotle (1 burrito bowl) = 705 cal

Carrots, Roasted Carrots, (1/2 cup) = 55 cal, (1 cup) = 110 cal

Calzone, Sausage w/cheese (1 calzone) = 1940 cal

Calzone, Ham w/cheese (1 calzone) = 1800 cal

Calzone, Vegetable w/cheese (1 calzone) = 1600 cal

Casserole, Tuna Casserole, (1 meal) = 344 cal

Chile, Beef chili (1 cup) = 170 cal

Chile, Veggie chili (1 cup) = 230 cal

Chimichanga, Beef (1 chimichanga) = 750 cal

Chimichanga, Chicken (1 chimichanga) = 700 cal

Corn (2/3 cup, frozen to cooked) = 80 cal

Corn on Cob (1 ear) = 83 cal

Corn Dog (1 corn dog) = 460 cal

Cornbread (1 piece) = 180 cal

Chicken Parmesan (1 serving) = 324 cal

Chicken, Breaded Chicken Cutlet (1 cutlet) = 300 cal

Chicken, Chicken Breast, skinless, cooked (1 cutlet) = 140 cal

Chicken, Chicken Katsu, fried, Japanese (1 katsu) = 332 cal

Chicken, Dijon Chicken (1 cutlet) = 178 cal

Chicken, Fried Chicken (1 piece) = 377 cal

Chicken, Grilled Chicken (3 oz) = 110 cal

Chicken, Lemon Herb Chicken (1 piece) = 190 cal

Chicken, Roast Chicken (3 oz) = 190 cal

Crab Cakes (2 med cakes) = 724 cal

MEALS

LUNCH / DINNER

Curry over Rice, Cauliflower Curry (1 cup curry, 1 cup rice) = 261 cal

Curry over Rice, Chicken Curry (1 cup curry, 1 cup rice) = 450 cal

Curry over Rice, Green Curry (1 cup curry, 1 cup rice) = 530 cal

Curry over Rice, Palak Paneer, Indian (1 cup curry, 1 cup rice) = 566 cal

Curry over Rice, Red Curry (1 cup curry, 1 cup rice) = 617 cal

Curry over Rice, Vegetable Curry (1 cup curry, 1 cup rice) = 522 cal

Deli Cheese, American cheese (1 slice) = 95 cal

Deli Cheese, Cheddar cheese (1 slice) = 113 cal

Deli Cheese, Jarlsberg cheese (1 slice) = 111 cal

Deli Cheese, Gouda cheese (1 slice) = 101 cal

Deli Cheese, Gruyere cheese (1 slice) = 116 cal

Deli Cheese, Manchebo cheese (1 slice) = 110 cal

Deli Cheese, Muenster cheese (1 slice) = 103 cal

Deli Cheese, Monterey Jack cheese (1 slice) = 106 cal

Deli Cheese, Mozzarella cheese (1 slice) = 78 cal

Deli Cheese, Pepper Jack cheese (1 slice) = 105 cal

Deli Cheese, Provolone cheese (1 slice) = 98 cal

Deli Cheese, Swiss Cheese (1 slice) = 106 cal

Deli Cheese, Swiss Cheese Light (1 slice) = 50 cal

Deli Meat, Chorizo, Spanish salami (1 slice) = 129 cal

Deli Meat, Corned Beef (1 slice) = 25 cal

Deli Meat, Ham, Black Forest (1 slice) = 70 cal

Deli Meat, Mortadella (1 slice) = 47 cal

Deli Meat, Pancetta, pork belly salami (1 thin slice) = 50 cal

Deli Meat, Pastrami (1 slice) = 41 cal

Deli Meat, Pepperoni (1 sm slice) = 20 cal

MEALS

Deli Meat, Prosciutto (1 slice) = 35 cal

Deli Meat, Roast Beef (1 slice) = 40 cal

Deli Meat, Salami (1 slice) = 41 cal

Deli Meat, Turkey (1 slice) = 28 cal

Egg Rolls, fried (1 egg roll) = 200 cal

Empanada, Beef (1 empanada) = 250 cal

Empanada, Chicken (1 empanada) = 299 cal

Enchiladas, Beef, cheese bean w/sauce (2 enchiladas) = 575 cal

Enchiladas, Cheese w/sauce (2 enchiladas) = 504 cal

Enchiladas, Chicken cheese bean w/sauce (2 enchiladas) = 540 cal

Fajitas, Chicken w/vegetables, toppings (2 fajitas) = 705 cal

Fajitas, Steak w/vegetables, toppings (2 fajitas) = 1565 cal

Fish & Chips, fried cod w/french fries (1 platter) = 800-1000 cal

Fish, Cod Baked (1 fillet) = 190 cal

Fish, Haddock Broiled or Baked, (1 med fillet) = 197 cal

Fish, Mahi Mahi, Grilled (1 fillet, steak sized) = 135 cal

Fish, Salmon Baked (1 fillet, 3oz) = 157 cal

Fish, Salmon Steamed (1 fillet, 3oz) = 157 cal

Fish, Salmon Pan-Fried (1 fillet, 3oz) = 187 cal

Fish, Swordfish, Grilled (1 fillet, steak sized) = 210 cal

Fish, Tilapia Baked (1 fillet) = 110 cal

Fish, Tuna, Grilled (1 fillet, steak sized) = 186 cal

Fish-Shellfish, Fisherman's Platter, fried seafood w/tartar sauce (1 platter) = 1900 cal

Fish-Shellfish, Clams Fried w/tartar sauce (20 sm clams) = 500 cal

Fish-Shellfish, Clams Steamed (12 sm clams) = 130 cal

MEALS

LUNCH / DINNER

Fish-Shellfish, Oysters Raw (3 oysters) = 130 cal

Fish-Shellfish, Oysters Fried (6 med oysters) = 400 cal

Fish-Scallops, Scallops Steamed (4 lg scallops) = 127 cal

Fish-Scallops, Scallops Pan-Fried w/butter (4-5 lg scallops) = 220 cal

Fish-Shellfish, Shrimps Fried (4 lg shrimps) = 152 cal

Fish-Shellfish, Shrimps Steamed (4 lg shrimps) = 26 cal

Fish-Shellfish, Lobster (1 med Maine lobster, flesh only) = 130 cal, (w/butter sauce) = 540 cal

French Fries, Fast food fries, (small fries) = 230 cal, (med fries) = 340 cal, (large fries) = 510 cal

French Fries, Oven Baked Fries, from frozen, (10 fries) = 99 cal

French Fries, Steak Cut fries, (10 fries) = 202 cal, (20 fries) = 404 cal

French Fries, Restaurant fries, (1 order) = 607 cal

Green Beans, sautéed (1/2 cup) = 50 cal, (1 cup) = 100 cal

Green Beans, steamed (1/2 cup) = 35 cal, (1 cup) = 70 cal

Green Peas, boiled w/salt (1/2 cup) = 67 cal, (1/2 cup) = 134 cal

Hot Dog, beef w/fixings (1 hotdog) = 284 cal

Mac & Cheese, homemade (1/2 cup) = 230 cal, (1 cup) = 460 cal

Meatloaf (1 slice) = 330 cal

Meatballs, Beef & Pork (3 meatballs) = 250 cal

Meatballs, Chicken Meatballs w/caramelized onions (3 meatballs) = 130 cal

Meatballs, Turkey meatballs (3 meatballs) = 150 cal

Meatballs, Veggie meatballs (3 meatballs) = 100 cal

Nachos, w/cheese fixings (1 order) = 1234 cal

Onion Rings, Beer Battered Onion Rings, at restaurant (1 order) = 1000 cal

Onion Rings, Home Onion Rings, from frozen (10 rings) = 280 cal

MEALS

LUNCH / DINNER

Onion Rings, Fast Food, (sm) = 320 cal, (med) = 410 cal, (lg) = 500 cal

Pad Thai (1 plate) = 838 cal

Pasta, Baked Ziti (1 cup) = 360 cal, (1 plate) = 760 cal

Pasta, Lasagna, Meat (1 square) = 600 cal

Pasta, Lasagna, Veggie (1 square) = 314 cal

Pasta, Spaghetti Bolognese (1 plate) = 800 cal

Pasta, Spaghetti with Meatballs (1 plate) = 800 cal

Pasta, Spaghetti with Pesto Sauce (1 plate) = 760 cal

Pasta, Spaghetti w/Chicken Parmesan (1 plate) = 862 cal

Pasta, Penne w/Chicken & Basil Pesto (1 plate) = 580 cal

Pasta, Penne w/Chicken & Broccoli (1 plate) = 510 cal

Pasta, Penne w/Italian Sausage & Pepper (1 plate) = 450 cal

Pasta, Penne Whole Wheat w/Chicken & Broccoli (1 plate) = 400 cal

Pizza, Plain slice (1 slice) = 285 cal

Pizza, Pepperoni slice (1 slice) = 380 cal

Pizza, Margherita Thin Crust Pizza (individual size) = 400 cal

Pork, Pork Cutlet Breaded (1 pork cutlet) = 460 cal

Pork, Pork Katsu, fried, Japanese (1 katsu) = 482 cal

Pork, Pork Sirloin (3 oz cut) = 163 cal

Pork, Pork Tenderloin (3 oz cut) = 135 cal

Potatoes, Baked Potato (1 baked potato) = 161 cal

Potatoes, Roasted Potatoes, red or yukon gold (1/2 cup) = 90 cal, (1 cup) = 180 cal

Potatoes, Mashed Potatoes, red or yukon gold w/milk, butter (1/2 cup) = 120 cal, (1 cup) = 240 cal

Quesadilla, Black bean & cheese (1 quesadilla, 8-10") = 710 cal

Quesadilla, Chicken w/cheese (1 quesadilla, 8-10") = 1069 cal

MEALS

LUNCH / DINNER

Quesadilla, Meat w/cheese (1 quesadilla, 8-10") = 1192 cal

Ramen, Beef w/egg, noodles (1 bowl) = 976 cal

Ramen, Shoyu Chicken w/egg, noodles (1 bowl) = 954 cal

Ramen, Tonkatsu Pork w/egg, noodles (1 bowl) = 660 cal

Ramen, Miso w/chicken, egg, noodles (1 bowl) = 596 cal

Ramen, Veggie, Homemade, Ginger (1 bowl) = 350 cal

Rice, Brown Rice, cooked (1/2 cup) = 108 cal, (3/4 cup) = 162 cal, (1 cup) = 216 cal

Rice, Fried Rice, fried in wok w/eggs, vegetables, meat or seafood (1 cup) = 228 cal

Rice, White Rice, Japanese sushi rice, cooked (1/2 cup) = 125 cal,
(3/4 cup) = 187 cal, (1 cup) = 250 cal

Rice, White Rice, Jasmine white rice, Thai, long grained, cooked
(1/2 cup) = 103 cal, (3/4 cup) = 160 cal, (1 cup) = 205 cal

Rice, White Rice, short grain, cooked (1/2 cup) = 103 cal, (3/4 cup)
= 153 cal, (1 cup) = 206 cal

Rice, Wild Rice, cooked (1/2 cup) = 83 cal, (3/4 cup) = 125 cal, (1 cup) = 166 cal

Rice Ball, Ume, Pickled Plum (1 rice ball) = 168 cal

Rice Ball, Salmon (1 rice ball) = 160 cal

Rice Ball, Tuna Onigiri (1 rice ball) = 200 cal

Rice Bowl, Beef Bowl w/white rice, Japanese (1 bowl) = 620 cal

Rice Bowl, Chicken Teriyaki w/white rice, Japanese (1 bowl) = 600 cal

Salad, Caesar Salad, caesar dressing, crouton, parmesan (1 bowl) = 460 cal

Salad, Chicken Caesar Salad, grilled chicken, caesar dressing, crouton, parmesan
(1 bowl) = 590 cal

Salad, Cobb Salad, grilled chicken, avocado, egg (1 bowl) = 600 cal

Salad, Garden Salad, Tossed salad w/veggies (1 bowl) = 84 cal

Salad, Greek Salad, w/feta, olives, veggies (1 bowl) = 360 cal

MEALS

LUNCH / DINNER

Salad, Potato Salad (1/3 cup) = 94 cal, (1 cup) = 358 cal

Salad, Tuna Salad (1/3 cup) = 156 cal, (1 cup) = 380 cal

Salad dressing, Balsamic Vinaigrette (2 tbsp) = 150 cal

Salad dressing, Balsamic Fat Free (2 tbsp) = 26 cal

Salad dressing, Caesar (2 tbsp) = 160 cal

Salad dressing, French (2 tbsp) = 146 cal

Salad dressing, Ranch (2 tbsp) = 142 cal

Salad dressing, Ranch Light (2 tbsp) = 120 cal

Salad dressing, Thousand Island (2 tbsp) = 130 cal

Sandwich, BLT (1 sandwich) = 370 cal

Sandwich, Grilled Chicken (1 sandwich) = 370 cal

Sandwich, Crispy Chicken (1 sandwich) = 520 cal

Sandwich, Chicken Salad on Whole Wheat (1 sandwich) = 423 cal

Sandwich, Fish Sandwich, fried w/tartar (1 sandwich) = 600 cal

Sandwich, Grilled Cheese (1 sandwich) = 400 cal

Sandwich, Ham & Swiss (1 sandwich) = 520 cal

Sandwich, Lobster Roll (1 sandwich) = 507 cal

Sandwich, Peanut Butter & Jelly (1 sandwich) = 810 cal

Sandwich, Sausage, Pepper & Onion in Roll (lg sausage roll) = 750 cal

Sandwich, Turkey & Swiss (1 sandwich) = 320 cal

Sandwich, Tomato, Mozzarella, Basil, French Bread (1 sandwich) = 488 cal

Sausage, Chicken Apple Sausage (1 link) = 180 cal

Sausage, Italian Sausage (1 link) = 260 cal

Sausage, Roasted Garlic Chicken Sausage, Trader Joe's (1 link) = 130 cal

Sausage, Roasted Garlic & Gruyere Sausage (1 link) = 190 cal

Sausage, Spinach & Feta Chicken Sausage, Trader Joe's (1 link) = 110 cal

MEALS

LUNCH / DINNER

Sausage, Portobello Mushroom & Swiss Cheese Chicken Sausage (1 link) = 180 cal

Sausage, Veggie Sausage (1 sausage) = 80 cal

Soup, Chicken Noodle Soup (1 cup) = 87 cal

Soup, Chicken Rice Soup (1 cup) = 60 cal

Soup, Clam Chowder, New England (1 cup) = 250 cal

Soup, Corn Chowder (1 cup) = 250 cal

Soup, Fish Soup (1 cup) = 105 cal, (1 bowl) = 210 cal

Soup, French Onion Soup w/fixings (1 crock) = 478 cal

Soup, Creamy Potato Soup (1 cup) = 200 cal

Soup, Tomato Bisque (1 cup) = 200 cal

Soup, Tomato Soup (1 cup) = 74 cal

Soup, Vegetable Soup (1 cup) = 80 cal

Steak, Beef Shoulder, roasted (3 oz Pot Roast) = 160 cal, (6 oz steak) = 320 cal

Steak, Beef Tenderloin or Filet Mignon, broiled (3 oz steak) = 230 cal, (6 oz steak) = 460 cal

Steak, Flank Steak, broiled (3 oz steak) = 160 cal, (6 oz steak) = 320 cal

Steak, Porterhouse, broiled (3 oz steak) = 180 cal, (6 oz steak) = 360 cal

Steak, Rib Eye, pan fried (3 oz steak) = 230 cal, (6 oz steak) = 470 cal

Steak, Skirt Steak, pan fried (3 oz steak) = 202 cal, (6 oz steak) = 404 cal

Steak, Steak Tips, grilled (3 steak tips) = 230 cal, (6 steak tips) = 460 cal

Steak, Top Sirloin, pan fried or grilled (3 oz steak) = 180 cal, (6 oz steak) = 360 cal

Steak, Tri Tip, grilled (3 oz steak) = 179 cal, (6 oz steak) = 358 cal

Stir Fry, Beef & Broccoli (1 cup) = 338 cal

Stir Fry, Chicken & Broccoli, garlic sauce (1 cup) = 219 cal

Stir Fry, Fried Rice (1 cup) = 300 cal (1 plate, restr) = 600 cal

Stir Fry, Ginger Chicken, garlic, soy (1 cup) = 300 cal

MEALS

LUNCH / DINNER

Stir Fry, Pork & Cabbage (1 cup) = 270 cal

Sub, Ham & Cheese Sub (6" sub) = 420 cal, (12" sub) = 840 cal

Sub, Italian Sub (6" sub) = 450 cal, (12" sub) = 900 cal

Sub, Meatball Sub w/Marinara (6" sub) = 480 cal, (12" sub) = 960 cal

Sub, Oven Roasted Chicken Sub (6" sub) = 320 cal, (12" sub) = 640 cal

Sub, Philly Cheese Steak (6" sub) = 600 cal, (12" sub) = 1146 cal

Sub, Pulled Pork (6" sub) = 455 cal, (12" sub) = 910 cal

Sub, Turkey Sub (6" sub) = 300 cal, (12" sub) = 600 cal

Sushi, Chirashi, sushi & vegetables on a bowl of rice (1 bowl) = 750 cal

Sushi, Roll (*raw fish or a sushi ingredient wrapped in a rice roll & seaweed*)

Sushi, Roll, Avocado Roll (per piece) = 25 cal, (6 pieces) = 140 cal

Sushi, Roll, California Roll (per piece) = 45 cal, (6 pieces) = 270 cal

Sushi, Roll, Caterpillar Roll, eel, fish roe, cucumber, avocado
(per piece) = 55 cal, (6 pieces) = 329 cal

Sushi, Roll, Dragon Roll (per piece) = 63 cal, (6 pieces) = 378 cal

Sushi, Roll, Eel Avocado Roll (per piece) = 62 cal, (6 pieces) = 372 cal

Sushi, Roll, Philadelphia Roll, salmon, cream cheese, avocado
(per piece) = 53 cal, (6 pieces) = 320 cal

Sushi, Roll, Rainbow Roll, mixed fish, veggies, avocado (per piece) = 79 cal,
(6 pieces) = 476 cal

Sushi, Roll, Salmon Roll (per piece) = 63 cal, (6 pieces) = 378 cal

Sushi, Roll, Salmon Avocado Roll (per piece) = 51 cal, (6 pieces) = 304 cal

Sushi, Roll, Shrimp Tempura Roll, shrimp, breaded, fried
(per piece) = 85 cal, (6 pieces) = 508 cal

Sushi, Roll, Spicy Tuna Roll, tuna, spicy mayo, hot sauce, green onions
(per piece) = 56 cal, (6 pieces) = 336 cal

MEALS

Sushi, Roll, Tuna Roll (per piece) = 31 cal, (6 pieces) = 184 cal

Sushi, Roll, Tuna Roll, set of 12 small rolls (per small piece) = 16 cal (12 pieces) = 260 cal

Sushi, Roll, Spider Roll, w/battered crab, avocado slices (per piece) = 53 cal, (6 pieces) = 317 cal

Sushi, Roll, Tempura Roll (per piece) = 66 cal, (6 pieces) = 396 cal

Sushi, Nigiri (*raw fish or a sushi ingredient on top of a bed of rice, usually à la carte or in mixed colorful platter of nigiri sushi*)

Sushi, Nigiri, Albacore Tuna (1 sushi) = 55 cal

Sushi, Nigiri, Eel (1 sushi) = 90 cal

Sushi, Nigiri, Egg Cake (1 sushi) = 73 cal

Sushi, Nigiri, Fish Roe (1 sushi) = 61 cal

Sushi, Nigiri, Mackerel, Saba (1 sushi) = 59 cal

Sushi, Nigiri, Octopus (1 sushi) = 57 cal

Sushi, Nigiri, Salmon (1 sushi) = 65 cal

Sushi, Nigiri, Salmon Roe, Ikura (1 sushi) = 65 cal

Sushi, Nigiri, Scallops (1 sushi) = 45 cal

Sushi, Nigiri, Sea Urchin (1 sushi) = 64 cal

Sushi, Nigiri, Shrimp, Ebi (1 sushi) = 44 cal

Sushi, Nigiri, Tuna (1 sushi) = 60 cal

Sushi, Nigiri, Yellowtail (1 sushi) = 54 cal

Sushi, Sashimi (*thinly sliced cut of raw fish that is served without rice*)

Sushi, Sashimi, Akami, Tuna, cheapest, most common cut of tuna, lean & very red, used often in rolls (1 sashimi) = 30 cal

Sushi, Sashimi, Amaebi, Sweet shrimp (1 sashimi) = 30 cal

Sushi, Sashimi, Awabi, Abalone (1 sashimi) = 30 cal

MEALS

Sushi, Sashimi, Burii, Yellowtail (1 sashimi) = 30 cal

Sushi, Sashimi, Hamachi, Japanese Amberjack/Yellowtail (1 sashimi) = 41 cal

Sushi, Sashimi, Hotate, Scallop (1 sashimi) = 39 cal

Sushi, Sashimi, Ika, Squid (1 sashimi) = 26 cal

Sushi, Sashimi, Ikura, Salmon Roe (1 sashimi) = 41 cal

Sushi, Sashimi, Kani, King Crab, steamed (1 sashimi) = 27 cal

Sushi, Sashimi, Kanpachi, Amberjack, type of Yellowtail (1 sashimi) = 41 cal

Sushi, Sashimi, Kantsuo, Bonito/Skipjack Tuna (1 sashimi) = 45 cal

Sushi, Sashimi, Maguro, Bluefish Tuna (1 sashimi) = 50 cal

Sushi, Sashimi, Saba, Mackerel (1 sashimi) = 58 cal

Sushi, (1 sashimi) = 70 cal

Sushi, Sashimi, Sake, Salmon (1 sashimi) = 50 cal

Sushi, Sashimi, Shiro Maguro, White Albacore Tuna (1 sashimi) = 49 cal

Sushi, Sashimi, Suzuki, Sea Bass (1 sashimi) = 41 cal

Sushi, Sashimi, Tai, Red Snapper, Sea Bream,(1 sashimi) = 22 cal

Sushi, Sashimi, Tako, Octopus (1 sashimi) = 53 cal

Sushi, Sashimi, Tamago, Japanese Omelet (1 sashimi) = 75 cal

Sushi, Sashimi, Uni, Sea Urchin (1 sashimi) = 40 cal

Tacos, Average Soft Taco w/meat filling (1 taco) = 200 cal

Tacos, Beef Tacos w/toppings (3 tacos) = 630 cal

Tacos, Chicken Tacos w/toppings (3 tacos) = 555 cal

Tacos, Fish Tacos w/toppings (3 tacos) = 600 cal

Tacos, Shredded Pork Tacos w/toppings (3 tacos) = 600 cal

Turkey, Deli Meat, Turkey (1 slice) = 25 cal

Turkey, Roast Turkey (3 oz) = 125 cal

MEALS

DESSERTS

Banana Bread (1 slice) = 196 cal

Brownie, homemade brownie (1 square) = 150 cal

Brownie, store brownie (1 square) = 250 cal

Cake, Angel Food Cake (1 piece) = 110 cal

Cake, Carrot Cake (1 piece) = 580 cal

Cake, Cheese Cake (1 piece) = 350 cal

Cake, Chocolate Cake (1 piece) = 400 cal

Cake, Pound Cake (1 piece) = 220 cal

Cake, Yellow Cake (1 piece) = 250 cal

Coffee Cake, w/crumb top (1 square) = 390 cal

Cookies, Chocolate Chip (1 cookie, 3″) = 80 cal, (lg cookie, 4″) = 221 cal

Cookies, Oatmeal Raisin (1 cookie, 3″) = 80 cal, (lg cookie, 4″) = 200 cal

Crepes, Banana Nutella Crepe (1 crepe) = 300 cal

Crepes, Buckwheat Crepe (1 crepe) = 100 cal

Crepes, Crepe w/Strawberry (1 crepe) = 182 cal

Crepes, Nutella Crepe (1 crepe) = 260 cal

Crepes, Plain Crepe (1 crepe) = 110 cal

Custard, Caramel Custard Flan (1 flan, 1/2 cup) = 260 cal

Cupcake, Chocolate Cupcake w/frosting (1 cupcake) = 473 cal

Cupcake, Coconut Cupcake w/frosting (1 cupcake) = 330 cal

Cupcake, Lemon Cupcake w/frosting (1 cupcake) = 330cal

Cupcake, Pumpkin Cupcake w/frosting (1 cupcake) = 304 cal

Cupcake, Red Velvet Cupcake w/frosting (1 cupcake) = 300 cal

Cupcake, Vanilla Cupcake w/frosting (1 cupcake) = 411 cal

Frozen Yogurt, most flavors (1/2 cup) = 110 cal, (1 cup) = 221 cal

Ice Cream, Chocolate (1 scoop) = 143 cal

MEALS

DESSERTS

Ice Cream, Coffee (1 scoop) = 137 cal

Ice Cream, Strawberry (1 scoop) = 127 cal

Ice Cream, Vanilla (1 scoop) = 137 cal

Ice Cream Bar, Coffee Almond Crunch Bar, Haagen-Daz (1 bar) = 290 cal

Ice Cream Bar, Ice Cream Sandwich (1 sandwich) = 166 cal

Ice Cream Sundae, Banana Split 3 scoops, syrup, all fixings (1 sundae) = 850-1000 cal

Ice Cream Sundae, Chocolate, 2 scoops, whp crm, all fixings (1 sundae) = 600 cal

Ice Cream Sundae, Vanilla Hot Fudge, 2 scoops, whp crm, all fixing (1 sundae) = 650 cal

Macaroons, Homemade (1 macaroon) = 97 cal

Macaroons, Coconut (1 macaroon) = 101 cal

Parfait, Homemade Parfait, yogurt/fruit/honey (1 parfait) = 150 cal

Parfait, Homemade Parfait, greek yogurt/berries/muesli (1 parfait) = 299 cal

Parfait, McDonald's Parfait, yogurt/fruit/granola (1 parfait) = 150 cal

Parfait, Starbuck's Parfait, greek yogurt/berries/granola (1 parfait) = 220 cal

Pastry, Cinnamon Bun (1 pastry) = 330 cal

Pastry, Danish (1 pastry) = 270 cal

Pie, Apple Pie, homemade (1 slice) = 360 cal

Pie, Banana Cream Pie, homemade (1 slice) = 325 cal

Pie, Blueberry Pie, homemade (1 slice) = 360 cal

Pie, Cherry Pie, homemade (1 slice) = 486 cal

Pie, Custard Pie, homemade (1 slice) = 222 cal

Pie, Key Lime Pie, homemade (1 slice) = 440 cal

Pie, Lemon Meringue Pie, homemade (1 slice) = 362 cal

Pie, Pecan Pie, homemade (1 slice) = 503 cal

Pie, Pumpkin Pie, homemade (1 slice) = 320 cal

Pie, Strawberry Rhubarb Pie, homemade (1 slice) = 422 cal

MEALS

DESSERTS

Pudding, Banana Pudding (1/2 cup) = 144 cal, (1 cup) = 288 cal

Pudding, Bread Pudding (1/2 cup) = 189 cal, (1 cup) = 377 cal

Pudding, Chocolate Pudding (1/2 cup) = 170 cal, (1 cup) = 340 cal

Pudding, Custard Pudding (1/2 cup) = 150 cal, (1 cup) = 300 cal

Pudding, Rice Pudding (1/2 cup) = 140 cal, (1 cup) = 280 cal

Pudding, Tapioca Pudding (1/2 cup) = 120 cal, (1 cup) = 240 cal

Tiramisu (1 dessert) = 450 cal

Whip Cream (2 tbsp) = 15 cal

MEALS

Avocado Toast, slice of toast with avocado spread (1 piece) = 200 cal

Applesauce, sweetened (1 cup) = 166 cal unsweetened (1 cup) = 50 cal

Bar, Chocolate, Dark Chocolate Bar (4 pieces) = 210 cal (1 bar) = 885 cal

Bar, Granola Bar (1 bar) = 120 cal

Bar, Protein Bar (1 bar) = 200 cal

Cheese & Water Crackers, w/mozzarella cheese (4 crackers, 1 oz cut Mozz) = 137 cal

Chips, Potato Chips (15 chips) = 140 cal

Chips, Tortilla Chips (10 chips) = 140 cal

Chips, Yellow Corn Chips (10 chips) = 130 cal

Cookie, Chocolate Chip (1 cookie, 3″) = 80 cal, (lg cookie, 4″) = 221 cal

Cookie, Oatmeal Raisin (1 cookie, 3″) = 80 cal, (lg cookie, 4″) = 200 cal

Crackers, Water Crackers (4 crackers) = 60 cal

Fig Newtons / Fig Bars (1 cookie) = 55 cal

Graham Crackers (2 full cracker sheets) = 130 cal

Graham Crackers, Lowfat (2 full cracker sheets) = 120 cal

Melba Toast (3 toasts) = 60 cal

Nuts, Almonds, raw (10 almonds) = 70 cal, (1/2 cup) = 238 cal, (1 cup) = 475 cal

Nuts, Mixed Nuts, roasted (10 nuts) = 86 cal, (1/2 cup) = 406 cal, (1 cup) = 693 cal

Nuts, Peanuts, roasted (10 peanuts) = 58 cal, (1/2 cup) = 414 cal, (1 cup) = 828 cal

Parfait, Homemade Parfait, yogurt/fruit/honey (1 parfait) = 125 cal

Parfait, McDonald's Parfait, yogurt/fruit/granola (1 parfait) = 150 cal

Parfait, Starbuck's Parfait, Greek yogurt/berries/granola (1 parfait) = 220 cal

Raisins, (sm box) = 130 cal (1/4 cup) = 130 cal, (1/2 cup) = 247 cal, (1 cup) = 494 cal

Salsa (1/2 cup) = 36 cal (1 cup) = 72 cal

String Cheese (1 mozzarella cheese stick) = 80 cal, Light = 50 cal

Trail Mix, w/raisins, nuts, seeds (1/2 cup) = 330 cal, (1 cup) = 813 cal

DRINKS

DRINKS & SMOOTHIES

Beer, Average Beer (12 oz, 1 bottle) = 153 cal

Beer, Amstel Light (1 bottle) = 95 cal

Beer, Corona Beer (1 bottle) = 154 cal

Beer, Coors Light Beer (1 bottle) = 102 cal

Beer, Guinness Draught Beer (12 oz, 1 bottle) = 125 cal

Beer, Harpoon Belgian Pale Ale (1 bottle) = 175 cal

Beer, Heineken (1 bottle) = 180 cal

Beer, Heineken Light (1 bottle) = 99 cal

Beer, Sierra Nevada Pale Ale (1 bottle) = 175 cal

Beer, Stella Artois (1 bottle) = 175 cal

Coffee, Black Coffee (1 cup) = 5 cal

Coffee, Cappuccino, milk froth, espresso (6oz cup) = 52 cal

Coffee, Coffee w/skim milk (1 cup) = 25 cal (w/skim milk & sugar) = 55 cal

Coffee, Coffee w/whole milk (1 cup) = 45 cal

Coffee, Espresso (1 shot) = 5 cal

Coffee, Iced Coffee (1 cup) = 5 cal, (1 cup w/skim milk) = 25 cal

Coffee, Latte (1 cup) = 136 cal

Coffee, Latte Nonfat, w/skim milk (1 cup) = 70 cal

Frappuccino, Starbucks, Tall size, milk, coffee syrup, sugar, ice, whipped cream (12 oz, Tall) = 300 cal

Juice, Apple Juice (1 cup) = 140 cal

Juice, Orange Juice (1 cup) = 110 cal

Juice, Orange Juice, Trop 50 (1 cup) = 50 cal

Shakes, Banana Ice Cream Milkshake, bananas, vanilla ice cream, milk, sugar (12 oz) = 452 cal

Shakes, Chocolate Ice Cream Milkshake, at fast food (12 oz) = 350-450 cal

DRINKS

DRINKS & SMOOTHIES

Shakes, Coffee Ice Cream Milkshake, at fast food or restaurants
(12 oz) = 350-450 cal

Shakes, Strawberry Ice Cream Milkshake, at fast food or restaurants
(12 oz) = 350-450 cal

Shakes, Vanilla Ice Cream Milkshake, at fast food or restaurants
(12 oz) = 350-450 cal

Smoothie, Banana Smoothie, banana, milk, brown sugar
(1 cup, homemade) = 176 cal, (16 oz, store size) = 352 cal

Smoothie, Banana Berry Smoothie, banana, berries, yogurt, honey, sugar
(1 cup, homemade) = 161 cal, (16 oz, store size) = 322 cal

Smoothie, Banana Mango Smoothie, banana, mango, yogurt, milk
(1 cup, homemade) = 140 cal, (16 oz, store size) = 280 cal

Smoothie, Green Smoothie, kale, apple, banana, oj, flax seed
(1 cup, homemade) = 123 cal, (16 oz, store size) = 246 cal

Smoothie, Kale Strawberry Banana Smoothie, kale, yogurt, strawberries,
honey, bananas, sugar (1 cup, homemade) = 189 cal, (16 oz, store size) = 378 cal

Smoothie, Mango Smoothie, mango, milk, vanilla yogurt, vanilla, ice
(1 cup, homemade) = 121 cal, (16 oz, store size) = 242 cal

Smoothie, Strawberry Smoothie, strawberries, skim milk, yogurt, sugar, vanilla
(1 cup, homemade) = 183 cal, (16 oz, store size) = 365 cal

Smoothie, Strawberry Banana Smoothie, strawberries, banana, yogurt, sugar, honey
(1 cup, homemade) = 161 cal, (16 oz, store size) = 322 cal

Smoothie, Tropical Smoothie, mango, papaya, strawberries, oj, sugar
(1 cup, homemade) = 126 cal, (16 oz, store size) = 252 cal

Soda, Coca-Cola, Coke (1 can) = 140 cal

Soda, Coca-Cola, Diet Coke (1 can) = 0 cal

DRINKS

DRINKS & SMOOTHIES

Soda, Carbonated Soda Water or Club Soda (1 can) = 0 cal

Soda, Pepsi-cola, Pepsi (1 can) = 150 cal

Soda, Pepsi-cola, Diet Pepsi (1 can) = 0 cal

Soda, Ginger Ale (1 can) = 140 cal

Tea, Iced Tea, Sweetened (1 cup) = 70 cal

Tea, Iced Tea, Unsweetened (1 cup) = 0 cal

Tea, Cold Tea, brewed, cold (1 cup) = 2 cal

Tea, Cold Tea, brewed, cold (1 cup + add milk & sugar) = 40 cal

Tea, Hot Tea, brewed, hot (1 cup) = 2 cal

Tea, Hot Tea, brewed, hot (1 cup + add milk & sugar) = 40 cal

Tea, Earl Grey Tea, brewed, hot (1 cup) = 2 cal

Tea, Green Tea, brewed, hot/cold (1 cup) = 2 cal

Water, Water regular, plain, tap or filtered (1 cup) = 0

Water, Water, carbonated (1 cup) = 0

Water, Water, sparkling (1 cup) = 0

Wine, Red Wine (5 fl oz glass) = 125 cal

Wine, Chardonnay Wine (5 fl oz glass) = 110 cal

Wine, Sake Rice Wine (1 fl oz) = 39 cal

Wine, White Wine (5 fl oz glass) = 121 cal

CONDIMENTS

CONDIMENTS

Almond Butter (1 tbsp) = 100 cal

Apple Butter (1 tbsp) = 30 cal

Applesauce (1 tbsp) = 11 cal

BBQ Sauce (1 tbsp) = 35 cal

Butter (1 tbsp) = 100 cal

Butter, Whipped Butter (1 tbsp) = 70 cal

Butter, Garlic Butter (1 tbsp) = 100 cal

Capers (1 tbsp) = 2 cal

Caramel (1 tbsp) = 50 cal

Chile Sauce (1 tbsp) = 20 cal

Chocolate Sauce (1 tbsp) = 55 cal

Chocolate Syrup (1 tbsp) = 55 cal

Cream Cheese (1 tbsp) = 50 cal

Cream Cheese. Light (1 tbsp) = 30 cal

Duck Sauce (1 tbsp) = 41 cal

Fish Sauce (1 tbsp) = 5 cal

Hot Sauce (1 tbsp) = 5 cal

Hot Sauce, Sriracha (1 tbsp) = 5 cal

Honey (1 tbsp) = 63 cal

Horseradish (1 tbsp) = 2 cal

Hot Peppers (1 tbsp) = 18 cal

Ginger, grounded (1 tbsp) = 5 cal

Guacamole (1 tbsp) = 30 cal

Hummus (1 tbsp) = 25 cal

Jalapeño Peppers (1 piece) = 4 cal

Jam, Blueberry (1 tbsp) = 50 cal

CONDIMENTS

CONDIMENTS

Jam, Strawberry (1 tbsp) = 56 cal

Ketchup (1 tbsp) = 20 cal

Lemon juice (1 tbsp) = 2 cal

Lime juice (1 tbsp) = 4 cal

Mango Chutney (1 tbsp) = 25 cal

Mayonnaise (1 tbsp) = 90 cal

Mayonnaise, Light (1 tbsp) = 35 cal

Maple Syrup (1 tbsp) = 52 cal

Mirin Cooking Wine (1 tbsp) = 50 cal

Mustard, Dijon (1 tbsp) = 5 cal

Mustard, Honey Mustard (1 tbsp) = 10 cal

Mustard, Yellow Mustard (1 tbsp) = 5 cal

Mustard, Whole seed (1 tbsp) = 10 cal

Nutella (1 tbsp) = 100 cal

Oil, Olive Oil (1 tbsp) = 120 cal

Oil, Sesame Oil (1 tbsp) = 120 cal

Olives (1 olive) = 5 cal

Peanut Butter (1 tbsp) = 100 cal

Pesto (1 tbsp) = 80 cal

Pickles (1 pickle) = 5 cal

Ranch Dressing (1 tbsp) = 72 cal

Ranch Dressing, Light (1 tbsp) = 56 cal

Relish (1 tbsp) = 20 cal

Roasted Red Peppers (1 piece) = 5 cal

Salsa, Chunky Salsa (1 tbsp) = 5 cal

Salsa, Picante Sauce (1 tbsp) = 1 cal

CONDIMENTS

CONDIMENTS

Salt (1 tsp) = 0 cal

Sesame Seeds (1 tbsp) = 52 cal

Sour Cream (1 tbsp) = 25 cal

Sour Cream, Light (1 tbsp) = 20 cal

Soy Sauce (1 tbsp) = 8 cal

Sriracha Hot Chili Sauce (1 tbsp) = 5 cal

Sugar (1 tbsp) = 16 cal

Sugar, pack (1 pack) = 20 cal

Sun-dried Tomatoes (1 piece) = 5 cal

Steak Sauce (1 tbsp) = 15 cal

Sweet & Sour Sauce (1 tbsp) = 30 cal

Tartar Sauce (1 tbsp) = 32 cal

Wasabi (1 tbsp) = 25 cal

Whipped Cream (1 tbsp) = 15 cal

Worcestershire sauce (1 tbsp) = 13 cal

Vanilla (1 tbsp) = 38 cal

Vinegar, Balsamic (1 tbsp) = 14 cal

Vinegar, Rice Vinegar (1 tbsp) = 3 cal

Vinegar, White (1 tbsp) = 3 cal

food groups

meat, poultry, eggs & fish

dairy, milk & cheese

breads

pasta, grains, & rice

vegetables

+ nuts & beans

fruits

FOOD GROUPS

MEAT, POULTRY, EGGS & FISH

BEEF

Beef, BBQ Ribs (1/2 rack, 6 ribs) = 762 cal

Beef, Brisket (3 oz) = 296 cal

Beef, Ground Beef, hamburger meat, sautéed, 80% lean (3 oz) = 200 cal

Beef, Hamburger Steak (1 serving) = 296 cal

Beef Stew, homemade, (1 cup) = 267 cal (1 bowl) = 535 cal

Burger, Cheeseburger w/toppings (reg size) = 400 cal, (lg size) = 550-700 cal

Burger, Hamburger w/toppings (reg size) = 300 cal, (lg size) = 400-500 cal

Deli Meat, Chorizo, Spanish salami (1 slice) = 129 cal

Deli Meat, Corned Beef (1 slice) = 25 cal

Deli Meat, Mortadella (1 slice) = 47 cal

Deli Meat, Pancetta, pork belly salami (1 thin slice) = 50 cal

Deli Meat, Pastrami (1 slice) = 41 cal

Deli Meat, Pepperoni (1 sm slice) = 20 cal

Deli Meat, Roast Beef (1 slice) = 40 cal

Deli Meat, Salami (1 slice) = 41 cal

Hot Dog, beef w/fixings (1 hotdog) = 284 cal

Sausage, Pepper & Onion in Roll (lg sausage roll) = 750 cal

Sausage, Italian Sausage (1 link) = 260 cal

Steak, Beef Shoulder, roasted (3 oz Pot Roast) = 160 cal, (6 oz steak) = 320 cal

Steak, Beef Tenderloin or Filet Mignon, broiled (3 oz steak) = 230 cal, (6 oz steak) = 460 cal

Steak, Flank Steak, broiled (3 oz steak) = 160 cal, (6 oz steak) = 320 cal

Steak, Porterhouse, broiled (3 oz steak) = 180 cal, (6 oz steak) = 360 cal

Steak, Rib Eye, pan fried (3 oz steak) = 230 cal, (6 oz steak) = 470 cal

Steak, Skirt Steak, pan fried (3 oz steak) = 202 cal, (6 oz steak) = 404 cal

Steak, Steak Tips, grilled (3 steak tips) = 230 cal, (6 steak tips) = 460 cal

FOOD GROUPS

MEAT, POULTRY, EGGS & FISH

Steak, Top Sirloin, pan fried or grilled (3 oz steak) = 180 cal, (6 oz steak) = 360 cal

Steak, Tri Tip, grilled (3 oz steak) = 179 cal, (6 oz steak) = 358 cal

Tacos, Average Soft Taco w/meat filling (1 taco) = 200 cal

Tacos, Beef Tacos w/toppings (3 tacos) = 630 cal

CHICKEN

Chicken Parmesan (1 serving) = 324 cal

Chicken, Breaded Chicken Cutlet (1 cutlet) = 300 cal

Chicken, Chicken Breast, skinless, cooked (1 cutlet) = 140 cal

Chicken, Chicken Katsu, fried, Japanese (1 katsu) = 332 cal

Chicken, Dijon Chicken (1 cutlet) = 178 cal

Chicken, Fried Chicken (1 piece) = 377 cal

Chicken, Grilled Chicken (3 oz) = 110 cal

Chicken, Lemon Herb Chicken (1 piece) = 190 cal

Chicken, Roast Chicken (3 oz) = 190 cal

Sandwich, Grilled Chicken (1 sandwich) = 370 cal

Sandwich, Crispy Chicken (1 sandwich) = 520 cal

Sandwich, Chicken Salad on Whole Wheat (1 sandwich) = 423 cal

Sausage, Chicken Apple Sausage (1 link) = 180 cal

Sausage, Roasted Garlic Chicken Sausage, Trader Joe's (1 link) = 130 cal

Sausage, Roasted Garlic & Gruyere Chicken Sausage (1 link) = 190 cal

Sausage, Spinach & Feta Chicken Sausage, Trader Joe's (1 link) = 110 cal

Sausage, Portobello Mushroom & Swiss Cheese Chicken Sausage (1 link) = 180 cal

Sausage, Breakfast Sausage, pork (3 sm links) = 180 cal

Soup, Chicken Noodle Soup (1 cup) = 87 cal

Soup, Chicken Rice Soup (1 cup) = 60 cal

FOOD GROUPS

MEAT, POULTRY, EGGS & FISH

EGGS

Eggs Benedict (2 eggs) = 553 cal

Eggs, Boiled (1 egg) = 78 cal

Eggs, Omelette, Ham & Cheese (2 eggs) = 300cal

Eggs, Omelette, Spinach, Mushroom, Tomato w/fresh fruit (2 eggs) = 330 cal

Eggs, Omelette, Veggies + Cheeses (2 eggs) = 495 cal

Eggs, Scrambled (1 egg) = 90 cal, (2 eggs) = 198 cal

Eggs, Sunnyside Up (1 egg) = 90 cal (2 eggs) = 180 cal

Egg Whites (3 tbsp = 1 egg) = 25 cal (6 tbsp = 2 eggs) = 50 cal

FISH & SEAFOOD

Crab Cakes (2 med cakes) = 724 cal

Fish & Chips, fried cod w/french fries (1 platter) = 800-1000 cal

Fish, Cod Baked (1 fillet) = 190 cal

Fish, Haddock Broiled or Baked, (1 med fillet) = 197 cal

Fish, Mahi Mahi, Grilled (1 fillet, steak sized) = 135 cal

Fish, Salmon Baked (1 fillet, 3oz) = 157 cal

Fish, Salmon Steamed (1 fillet, 3oz) = 157 cal

Fish, Salmon Pan-Fried (1 fillet, 3oz) = 187 cal

Fish, Swordfish, Grilled (1 fillet, steak sized) = 210 cal

Fish, Tilapia Baked (1 fillet) = 110 cal

Fish, Tuna, Grilled (1 fillet, steak sized) = 186 cal

Fish-Shellfish, Fisherman's Platter, fried seafood w/tartar sauce (1 platter) = 1900 cal

Fish-Shellfish, Clams Fried w/tartar sauce (20 sm clams) = 500 cal

Fish-Shellfish, Clams Steamed (12 sm clams) = 130 cal

Fish-Shellfish, Oysters Raw (3 oysters) = 130 cal

FOOD GROUPS

MEAT, POULTRY, EGGS & FISH

Fish-Shellfish, Oysters Fried (6 med oysters) = 400 cal

Fish-Scallops, Scallops Steamed (4 lg scallops) = 127 cal

Fish-Scallops, Scallops Pan-Fried w/butter (4-5 lg scallops) = 220 cal

Fish-Shellfish, Shrimps Fried (4 lg shrimps) = 152 cal

Fish-Shellfish, Shrimps Steamed (4 lg shrimps) = 26 cal

Fish-Shellfish, Lobster (1 med Maine lobster, flesh only) = 130 cal,
(w/butter sauce) = 540 cal

Sandwich, Fish Sandwich, fried w/tartar (1 sandwich) = 600 cal

Sandwich, Lobster Roll (1 sandwich) = 507 cal

Soup, Clam Chowder, New England (1 cup) = 250 cal

Soup, Fish Soup (1 cup) = 105 cal, (1 bowl) = 210 cal

Sushi, Chirashi, sushi & vegetables on a bowl of rice (1 bowl) = 750 cal

Sushi, Roll, Salmon Roll (per piece) = 63 cal, (6 pieces) = 378 cal

Sushi, Roll, Tuna Roll (per piece) = 31 cal, (6 pieces) = 184 cal

Sushi, Nigiri, Salmon (1 sushi) = 65 cal

Sushi, Nigiri, Tuna (1 sushi) = 60 cal

Sushi, Nigiri, Yellowtail (1 sushi) = 54 cal

Sushi, Sashimi, Sake, Salmon (1 sashimi) = 50 cal

PORK/HAM

Deli Meat, Ham, Black Forest (1 slice) = 70 cal

Deli Meat, Prosciutto (1 slice) = 35 cal

Pork, Pork Cutlet Breaded (1 pork cutlet) = 460 cal

Pork, Pork Katsu, fried, Japanese (1 katsu) = 482 cal

Pork, Pork Sirloin (3 oz cut) = 163 cal

Pork, Pork Tenderloin (3 oz cut) = 135 cal

FOOD GROUPS

MEAT, POULTRY & FISH

Sandwich, BLT bacon, lettuce, tomato, mayo (1 sandwich) = 370 cal

Sandwich, Ham & Swiss (1 sandwich) = 520 cal

TURKEY

Deli Meat, Turkey (1 slice) = 28 cal

Sandwich, Turkey & Swiss (1 sandwich) = 320 cal

Turkey, Deli Meat, Turkey (1 slice) = 25 cal

Turkey, Roast Turkey (3 oz) = 125 cal

Sausage, Turkey Sausage (3 sm links) = 100 cal

FOOD GROUPS

DAIRY, MILK & CHEESE

Cheese, American Cheese (1 slice) = 95 cal

Cheese, Brie Cheese (1 oz) = 100 cal

Cheese, Blue Cheese (1 oz) = 100 cal

Cheese, Cheddar Cheese (1 slice) = 113 cal   (1 oz wedge) = 115 cal

Cheese, Cream Cheese, Regular (1 tbsp) = 50 cal, (1/2 cup) = 397 cal

Cheese, Cream Cheese, Low-Fat (1 tbsp) = 30 cal, (1/2 cup) = 242 cal

Cheese, Cream Cheese, Whipped (1 tbsp) = 25 cal, (1/2 cup) = 200 cal

Cheese, Cream Cheese, Fat Free (1 tbsp) = 20 cal, (1/2 cup) = 138 cal

Cheese, Gruyere Cheese (1 slice) = 116 cal

Cheese, Mozzarella Cheese (1 slice/oz) = 80 cal (1/4 cup shredded) = 90 cal

Cheese, Mozzarella Cheese, Part Skim (1 slice/oz) = 70 cal (1/4 cup shredded) = 80 cal

Cheese, Provolone Cheese (1 slice) = 98 cal

Cheese, Ricotta Cheese (1 oz) = 60 cal

Cheese, Swiss Cheese (1 slice) = 106 cal, Light = 50 cal

Cottage Cheese (1 tbsp) = 20 cal, (1/2 cup) = 111 cal, (1 cup) = 222 cal

Cottage Cheese, Fat Free (1/2 cup) = 53 cal, (1 cup) = 105 cal

Cream, Heavy Cream (1 tbsp) = 52 cal, (1/2 cup) = 411 cal

Ice Cream, Vanilla (1 scoop) = 137 cal, Chocolate = 143 cal

Milk, 1% Low-fat Milk (1/3 cup) = 30 cal, (1/2 cup) = 51 cal, (1 cup) = 102 cal

Milk, 2% Low-fat Milk (1/3 cup) = 46 cal, (1/2 cup) = 69 cal, (1 cup) = 137 cal

Milk, Chocolate Milk (1/3 cup) = 70 cal, (1/2 cup) = 105 cal, (1 cup) = 209 cal

Milk, Nonfat or Skim Milk (1/3 cup) = 36 cal, (1/2 cup) = 51 cal, (1 cup) = 102 cal

Milk, Whole Milk (1/3 cup) = 49 cal, (1/2 cup) = 73 cal, (1 cup) = 148 cal

Yogurt, Plain (1 cup) = 90-110 cal, w/fruit = 110-150 cal

Yogurt, Greek Yogurt, Plain (1 cup) = 100-130 cal, w/fruit = 110-140 cal

Yogurt, Light, Non Fat Yogurt (1 cup) = 80-110 cal, w/fruit = 100-120 cal

FOOD GROUPS

BREADS

Bagel, plain (1 med bagel) = 250 cal

Baguette, French Baguette (6″ baguette) = 277 cal

Bread, Ciabatta (1 slice) = 100 cal, (2 slices) = 200 cal

Bread, French Bread (1 slice) = 88 cal, (2 slices) = 174 cal

Bread, Italian Bread (1 slice) = 80 cal, (2 slices) = 160 cal

Bread, Sourdough Bread (1 slice) = 110 cal, (2 slices) = 220 cal

Bread, White Bread (1 slice) = 60 cal, (2 slices) = 120 cal

Bread, Whole Wheat Bread (1 slice) = 68 cal, (2 slices) = 136 cal

Bread Rolls, Deli-Style Soft Roll (1 roll) = 170 cal

Bread Rolls, Dinner Roll (1 roll) = 129 cal

Bread Rolls, Hamburger Bun (1 roll) = 150 cal

Bread Rolls, Hot Dog Bun (1 roll) = 150 cal

Bread Rolls, Portuguese Roll (1 roll) = 220 cal

Bread Rolls, Sub Roll, white (6″ sub roll) = 200 cal

Bread Rolls, Sub Roll, whole wheat (6″ sub roll) = 180 cal

Cornbread (1 slice) = 180 cal

Croissant, Plain Butter (1 croissant) = 230 cal

Croissant, Chocolate (1 croissant) = 340 cal

Croissant, Almond (1 croissant) = 420 cal

Croissant, Ham & Swiss Cheese (1 croissant) = 320 cal

English Muffin Bread, toasted (1 muffin) = 130 cal, (2 muffins) = 260 cal

Naan Bread, Indian (1 piece naan) = 247 cal

Pita, Pita White Bread (1 pita, 6″) = 165 cal

Pita, Pita Whole Wheat Pita Bread (1 pita, 6″) = 170 cal

Rye Bread (1 slice) = 83 cal, (2 slices) = 166 cal

FOOD GROUPS

PASTA, RICE & GRAINS

Quinoa, cooked (3/4 cup) = 166 cal, (1 cup) = 222 cal

Pasta, Penne, cooked (1 cup) = 200 cal

Pasta, Penne whole wheat, cooked (1 cup) = 145 cal

Pasta, Linguini, cooked (1 cup) = 213 cal

Pasta, Macaroni elbow, cooked (1 cup) = 221 cal

Pasta, Macaroni elbow, whole wheat, cooked (1 cup) = 174 cal

Pasta, Shells, cooked (1 cup) = 156 cal

Pasta, Spaghetti, cooked (1 cup) = 221 cal

Pasta, Spaghetti whole-wheat, cooked (1 cup) = 174 cal

Rice, Brown Rice, cooked (1/2 cup) = 108 cal, (3/4 cup) = 162 cal, (1 cup) = 216 cal

Rice, White Rice, Japanese sushi rice, cooked (1/2 cup) = 125 cal, (3/4 cup) = 187 cal, (1 cup) = 250 cal

Rice, White Rice, Jasmine white rice, Thai, long grained, cooked (1/2 cup) = 103 cal, (3/4 cup) = 160 cal, (1 cup) = 205 cal

Rice, White Rice, short grain, cooked (1/2 cup) = 103 cal, (3/4 cup) = 153 cal, (1 cup) = 206 cal

Rice, Wild Rice, cooked (1/2 cup) = 83 cal, (3/4 cup) = 125 cal, (1 cup) = 166 cal

Rice Cake (1 rice cake) = 35 cal

FOOD GROUPS

VEGETABLES (+ NUTS & BEANS)

Almonds (1 cup) = 825 cal

Arugula (1 cup) = 3 cal

Artichoke (1 cup) = 89 cal

Asparagus (1 cup) = 27 cal

Avocado (1/2 cup) = 117 cal (1 fruit) = 322 cal

Beans, Baked Beans, cooked(1 cup) = 392 cal

Beans, Black Beans, cooked (1 cup) = 227 cal

Beans, Chickpeas, cooked (1 cup) = 269 cal

Beans, Fava Beans, cooked (1 cup) = 187 cal

Beans, Green Beans, cooked (1 cup) = 35 cal

Beans, Lentil Beans, cooked (1 cup) = 230 cal

Beans, Navy/White beans, cooked (1 cup) = 255 cal

Beans, Pinto Beans, cooked (1 cup) = 245 cal

Beans, Refried Beans, cooked (1 cup) = 218 cal

Beans, Soybeans, cooked (1 cup) = 254 cal

Beets (1 cup) = 59 cal

Bell Peppers (1 cup) = 40 cal

Bitter Melon (1 cup) = 20 cal

Bok Choy (1 cup) = 9 cal

Broccoli (1 cup) = 31 cal

Brussel Sprouts (1 cup) = 38 cal

Butternut Squash (1 cup) = 63 cal

Cabbage (1 cup) = 22 cal

Carrots (1 cup) = 53 cal

Cauliflower (1 cup) = 25 cal

Celery (1 cup) = 18 cal

FOOD GROUPS

VEGETABLES (+ NUTS & BEANS)

Chives (1 cup) = 14 cal

Collard Greens (1 cup) = 11 cal

Corn (1 cup) = 133 cal

Cucumber (1 cup) = 16 cal

Eggplant (1 cup) = 20 cal

Endive (1 cup) = 8 cal

Fennel (1 cup) = 27 cal

Garlic (1 clove) = 5 cal

Green Beans (1 cup) = 35 cal

Jicama (1 cup) = 46 cal

Kale (1 cup) = 34 cal

Onions (1 cup) = 46 cal

Leeks (1 cup) = 32 cal

Lemongrass (1 cup) = 66 cal

Lettuce (1 cup) = 5 cal

Mint leaves (2 leaves) = 1 cal

Mushrooms (1 cup) = 16 cal

Mustard Greens (1 cup) = 15 cal

Nuts, Brazil Nuts (1 cup) = 813 cal

Nuts, Cashews (1 cup) = 787 cal

Nuts, Macadamia (1 cup) = 962 cal

Nuts, Mixed Nuts (1 cup) = 813 cal

Nuts, Pecans (1 cup) = 684 cal

Nuts, Peanuts (1 cup) = 828 cal

Nuts, Pine Nuts (1 cup) = 909 cal

Nuts, Pistachio (1 cup) = 691 cal

Nuts, Walnuts (1 cup) = 523 cal

Okra (1 cup) = 33 cal

Parsnip (1 cup) = 100 cal

Peas (1 cup) = 118 cal

Peppers (1 cup) = 46 cal

Potatoes (1 cup) = 116 cal

Pumpkin (1 cup) = 30 cal

Radicchio (1 cup) = 9 cal

Radishes (1 cup) = 19 cal

Scallions (1 cup) = 32 cal

Shallots (1 shallot) = 31 cal

Snow Peas (1 cup) = 60 cal

Spinach (1 cup) = 7 cal

Sweet Potato (1 cup) = 114 cal

Swiss Chard (1 cup) = 7 cal

Tomatoes (1 cup) = 27 cal

Tomatillo (1 cup) = 42 cal

Turnip (1 cup) = 36 cal

White Mushrooms (1 cup) = 15 cal

Watercress (1 cup) = 4 cal

Wheatgrass (3 fl oz juice) = 20 cal

Yams (1 cup) = 177 cal

Yellow Squash (1 cup) =68 cal

Zucchini (1 cup) = 20 cal

FOOD GROUPS

FRUITS

Acai Berry (100gr puree packet) = 70 cal

Avocado (1/2 cup) = 117 cal (1 fruit) = 322 cal

Blackcurrants (1 cup) = 70 cal

Blueberries (1 cup) = 85 cal

Boysenberries (1 cup) = 66 cal

Breadfruit, raw (1 cup) = 226 cal

Cantaloupe (1 cup) = 60 cal

Cherries (1 cup) = 77 cal

Clementines (1 fruit) = 35 cal

Coconut (1 cup, shredded) = 283 cal

Cranberries, raw (1 cup) = 51 cal

Dates (1 cup) = 480 cal

Dragon Fruit (1 fruit) = 61 cal

Figs (1 fig) = 40 cal

Grapes (1 cup) = 62 cal

Grapefruit (1 fruit) = 102 cal

Guava (1 cup) = 112 cal

Honeydew Melon (1 cup) = 61 cal

Jackfruit (1 cup) = 157 cal

Kiwi (1 fruit) = 42 cal

Kumquats (1 fruit) = 13 cal

Lemon (1 tbsp juice) = 2 cal

Lime (1 tbsp juice) = 4 cal

Mango (1 cup) = 100 cal (1 fruit) = 200 cal

Nectarine (1 cup) = 63 cal

Olive (1 olive) = 5 cal (10 olives) = 60 cal

FOOD GROUPS

FRUITS

Orange (1 fruit) = 62 cal

Papaya (1 cup) = 55 cal

Pears (1 fruit) = 100 cal

Peach (1 cup) = 61 cal

Persimmons (1 fruit) = 32 cal

Pineapple (1 cup) = 82 cal

Plum (1 fruit) = 30 cal

Pomegranate (1/2 cup seeds/jce) = 72 cal

Raisins (1 cup) = 494 cal

Raspberries (1 cup) = 65 cal

Rhubarb (1 cup) = 26 cal

Strawberries (1 cup) = 54 cal

Tangerine (1 fruit) = 47 cal

Watermelon (1 cup) = 46 cal

Winter Melon (1 cup) = 17 cal

Yuzu (1 tbsp juice) = 6 cal

Vanilla (1 vanilla pod) = 2 cal (1 tsp) = 12 cal

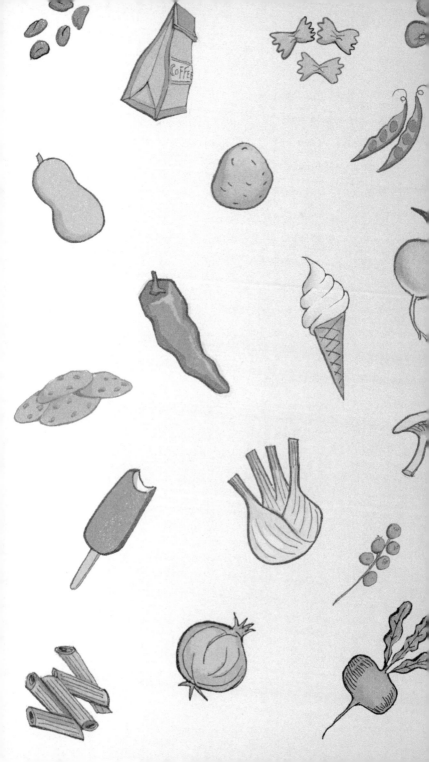

Printed in Great Britain
by Amazon